Do You Believe in Miracles?

Benetta Wainman

First published by Busybird Publishing 2016
Copyright © 2016 Benetta Wainman

ISBN
Print: 978-0-9953835-7-9
Ebook: 978-0-9953835-8-6

Benetta Wainman has asserted her right under the Copyright, Designs and Patents Act 1988 to be identified as the author of this work. The information in this book is based on the author's experiences and opinions. The publisher specifically disclaims responsibility for any adverse consequences, which may result from use of the information contained herein. Permission to use information has been sought by the author. Any breaches will be rectified in further editions of the book.

All rights reserved. No part of this publication may be reproduced, stored in or introduced into a retrieval system, or transmitted in any form, or by any means (electronic, mechanical, photocopying, recording or otherwise) without the prior written permission of the author. Any person who does any unauthorised act in relation to this publication may be liable to criminal prosecution and civil claims for damages. Enquiries should be made through the publisher.

Cover image: Kev Howlett
Cover design: Busybird Publishing
Layout and typesetting: Busybird Publishing
Editor: Jodie Garth

Busybird Publishing
PO Box 855
Eltham Victoria
Australia 3095
www.busybird.com.au

This book is dedicated to Shane and Jess Fozard for teaching me many skills in my profession as a hypnotherapist, and to my hypnosis family whom I thank God for every day, as they keep me sane in a sometimes insane world.

I could not have written this book, and indeed may not have carried on to become a hypnotherapist, without my family, friends and clients, who believed in me and let me practise on them when I really needed it. I love you all.

Contents

Foreword   i

Introduction   v

Part One   1

Chapter 1
  Look into my Eyes!   3

Chapter 2
  The Lightbulb Moment   7

Chapter 3
  Frequently Asked Questions   11

Chapter 4
  Is hypnotherapy magic or magical?   23

Part Two   35

Chapter 5
  Short and Sweet   37
    Anne-Marie's story   38
    Bethan's story   42
    Emily's story   44
    Linda's story   47
    Georgina's story   49
    Scott's story   53

Chapter 6
  OMG   57
    Jasmine's story   59
    Susie's story   63
    Teneil's story   68
    Here is Tina and Theo's story: 73

Chapter 7
  Conclusion   81

About the Author   83
Special Offer   85
Recommended Practitioners   87
Shane and Jess   92
Adair   93
Joy   95

Foreword

Is hypnotherapy becoming something that we, in the 21st century, are able to use as the new 'cure all'? I think the answer could be yes, if more people knew about it and believed that it worked.

Why I say this is that some of the things that I have witnessed with my own eyes, and seen in my own clients, is nothing short of amazing – mini miracles, in fact. This is why, in my capacity as a hypnotherapist, I felt compelled to write this book. I could have just taken the easier path, stopping people from smoking or helping them to lose weight (what I consider my 'bread and butter' in my work) and feeling good about myself for maybe helping them to not die from cancer or be debilitated by the fact that they, in a few years, would have been unable to live a productive and healthy life unless they decided to change those habitual ways.

Yes, I would have saved myself many hours at the computer and thousands of dollars self-funding this project, but would it have had an impact on thousands of people, opening their eyes to possibilities that they would otherwise have dismissed as impossible? My passion may just become yours or, at least, you can see how hypnotherapy helped me and how it can help you! That is, if you give it a chance because who knows what could happen if you believe in miracles as I now do. Even sceptics can be convinced, and this is my intent when writing this book.

This book is about giving you a taste of what hypnotherapy is and how it works. I will address some frequently asked questions and provide a few wonderful stories from real people, people like you and me, who just thought, 'What if?' or 'What do I have to lose?' or, more importantly, 'What do I have to gain if this does work?'

I now know that the possibilities are endless and if someone says to me, 'Have you treated this condition before?' I may have to say no, but that doesn't mean that I can't or that it is impossible. It just means that I have to put on my thinking cap a bit more on what to say to convince their subconscious that this is a really good idea and use some convincing words to show how this could work to get them moving in the right direction to obtain the outcome they want.

I say 'want', and want is good. If we can include 'need' then even better, as sometimes the things we want and need can be completely different. Someone once came to me and said that she wanted to lose weight. From where I was sitting she certainly did not need to lose any weight. She was drop dead gorgeous as well! 'Why does she need my services?' I asked myself, but looking deeper than the surface, I saw that her self-esteem was what was missing. She came to see me several times, too, and I could see a subtle change each time. Even though she did drop a few kilograms, which made her happy, she became stronger on the inside. She was able to deal with other issues much more easily, and was more relaxed and calm. Things are not always what they seem, are they?

When it comes to physical problems, it may be difficult to decipher which came first – the chicken or the egg. Could it have been that the brain decided something and then the physical problem materialised, or maybe that something physical started off a chain reaction which the brain ran with, and then the physical problem stayed even after it should have disappeared? If you are not following me too well here that is okay, because all will be revealed, just like a magician who seems to have magical powers; however, when the way in which the trick is done is then revealed, it all makes perfect sense.

Well, that is the object of this book. I truly hope that you think that it was worth my time, effort and money. You see, if I can help just a handful of people to change their lives for the better, then it will be worth it. If I can help a hundred, even better but what I really want is for thousands to do so. I want people all over the world to just try hypnotherapy and give it a chance, because who knows where it will lead? Do you?

Let this book lead you to a better, more fulfilling life – one that you never thought could be achieved through hypnotherapy and, just maybe, we can change the world, one person at a time. Come with me on a magical journey of discovery and together we can bring about the change that you have been searching for!

Introduction

Why did I start writing this book? I have asked myself this numerous times, especially when things weren't always going to plan or when I could be doing other things. Why did I even become a hypnotherapist in my late fifties after working as a nurse for most of my working life?

To be honest, I had been looking at something more holistic for a while. I couldn't work out why the medical profession would just want to medicate people for just about everything. Why was it that, instead of treating the cause, we were somehow treating the symptoms? I think I was pushed even further down this road when my son was started on medication for depression.

I saw overweight people being given drugs for high blood pressure, instead of putting them on a diet and exercise plan. It was all seeming too crazy.

Then I start thinking about it more and more and decided to see if there was something that I could do. I went on a course about hypnotherapy and loved everything about it. Then I went on a business seminar where I learned a lot, but then a man came out and said that we should write a book, and I felt a compelling need to write one from the time that I went to the seminar.

There was one problem: he wanted $40,000 for us to do it! He told us that we should because we would be seen as special being an author. Well, it wasn't that I wanted my name in print, looking special or that I would be seen as an expert in the field, which were ideas put into our minds when looking at writing a book. For me, it was purely and simply that I knew my profession as a hypnotherapist could be life-changing for many people and I wanted as many people as possible to try it out.

Prior to this, I'd had many strange responses from people about my profession – some thought it weird, some thought I would make them dance around making chicken sounds, but most were fearful that I would control their mind. Well, if they meant that they might somehow think in a different way, they would be right. If you think that buying blueberries instead of chocolate is crazy, when only minutes ago you told me that you wanted to swap chocolate for fruit to help you shed those excess kilograms, which just hasn't happened before, then I suppose it is. What you need to understand, however, is that this is really your decision and I have just helped your unconscious understand that you can do this.

I believe that I have found the best thing since sliced bread (I don't even like sliced bread myself much, as I am a cut-it-myself sort of girl), and I really think everyone should try it. Maybe reading the stories within this book will help you to see this. I am also including at the back of the book details of my website where you will be able to download a session to help you relax. It is great to listen to at the end of a long and tiring day, or to give you a break from what may be giving you a hard time.

I hope by giving you a little taste of hypnotherapy you will want more and see what I see, and feel how my clients feel when they leave my room. It may just be the miracle that you have been waiting for.

I was told to always work with an avatar in mind – my perfect client – and I just can't seem to do that. I find it very hard to choose between the man with Irritable Bowel Syndrome who has found life very difficult since he was in his teens, and the young girl with her life going nowhere good, or the 73-year-old who was molested as a 5-year-old and had a boulder on her chest that she couldn't ever think of getting rid of, or the young man with far too much on his plate … and the list goes on and on. Maybe one day I will specialise in something specific, but for now I have to say that my 'avatar' is anyone.

So, with this in mind, this book is directed at you, whoever you are and whatever your problem. I can't say that this problem will just disappear, but it might. I can't say that it will be an overnight thing, but it might be. What I can say is, let us work on it, and you may just have found the solution – you may have found that miracle that I am talking about, just as many have before you.

It may be that you live just around the corner from me in Diamond Creek, but it could be that even though you are reading my book, you are far away. Either way, we can work through it. We can Skype, I can write a session that you can listen to at home, or I can put you in touch with another hypnotherapist through my training group but, believe me, there is a way.

The first thing I will ask you, though, is 'How much does solving the problem mean to you?' On a scale of 1 to 10, I would like your score to be higher than a 5 out of 10. Why? Well, it would bring the best and biggest change to your life, and because this is what I want – to help you to change your life. Choosing something you may have tried to change many times before is even better – the bigger the change, the better.

When I was at my last training course, I was packing my suitcase to come back home and said to my friend of a week (now one of my besties), 'How weird – I seem to have less baggage than when I came. How about you?' She laughed, as when you do this hypnotherapy course, it is not all about learning new techniques (although we do, of course) but we practise on each other and so we come back solving our own problems too. So I did come back with much less baggage; we all did.

The week starts off with many glum faces (not everyone is there to become hypnotherapists as I was) and a sense of solitude. When the week ends, everyone is much more open, loud and free. I would encourage every single person to do these hypnotherapy courses. Everyone can get something out of them, and for many, like myself, it will change your life!

For now, however, come with me on a magical journey of discovery. Discover what hypnotherapy can do for you!

Part One

Chapter 1
Look into my Eyes!

I have found that when people first hear that I am a hypnotherapist they have a generalised misconception that I try and make people do obscure things like act like a chicken or do things they don't want to do. It may also include swinging a pendulum and saying things like 'Look into my eyes.' We can thank the stage hypnotist or the sensationalism of television or films for this view of hypnotherapy.

All stage hypnosis is performed by someone who is trained as a hypnotherapist, however, and I happened to be talking to one when I went to a 2-day course on how to write a book. He told me that he still does work as a hypnotherapist, helping people with such things as stopping smoking. I wondered how people still believed in his ability once they had seen him on stage. He said that his stage name and persona were completely separated and so people didn't know that he had a stage act. He sometimes even incorporated people's desires to change into his act. After meeting him I decided that those two sides of him were not that different, and my views on stage hypnosis changed quite a lot.

So, what is hypnosis? It is just a form of deep relaxation. I don't know if you have ever done any meditation ... if so, it is very similar. This 'hypnosis' is in order to talk to your unconscious mind, helping to activate the part of the brain that helps you to achieve your goals. All this means, though, is that you are in a totally relaxed state. You can hear, your conscious mind can follow or just go off in another direction, thinking about what is for dinner or whatever it wants.

This usually happens at the beginning of the hypnosis but tends to calm more as the relaxation goes on. The hypnotherapist has no intention to control your mind, or tell you to do things that you do not want to do. All that is taking place is to inform your unconscious brain that you have a problem and here is how to solve it. Each session is unique and tailored to the individual's traits and desire to resolve the problem and to improve the client's life.

The therapy side can also help you see why

you have not achieved your goals in the past by helping to unravel previous experiences and mental blocks. I want you to see that many, many things can be achieved with hypnotherapy. Some of the things that I have helped people with include smoking, weight loss and control, stress and anxiety, phobias, accelerated learning (especially year 12), getting a job or promotion, alcohol cessation or toning it down, self-confidence and habit control.

I do not intend to go into the techniques too much in this small book. This book will be mainly story-based as I want to share some clients' stories to show how they felt, their experiences and their results rather than techniques and statistics. Many of the people whom I see are using me as their last resort, the last chance to reach their goal. What I really would rather is for people to see me as their first port of call, the therapy they try first, not last.

Hypnotherapy changed my life, not because I now have thousands of dollars floating around, but because I know that *anything* is possible. I know that our minds are wonderful and incredible, but can also hold onto some crap too. Some things that should have been deleted but instead have been stored – stories that are untrue, or were once true but, now that time has passed, so should the issue.

This is a problem for many people. It could be that they started something like drinking heavily or smoking for pleasure to begin with, or to support them with a stressful time and then the stressful time passes but the drinking or smoking continues, becoming a habit. Pain is another problem that passes but the mind gets used to it and so it continues even when the pain should be long gone. The subconscious mind is a very convoluted, complicated and sometimes strange part of us, but its responsibility to keep us happy, healthy and safe, makes it easily changed if enough evidence is given in favour of the change. Read on to find out more if you are as intrigued as I had been.

Chapter 2
The Lightbulb Moment

For hypnotherapy to really work there are two real factors involved. Firstly, does the client really want the outcome? You might say, 'Of course, they must do as they have come to you for a change.' This may be so, but is it really important to them? On a scale of 1-10, how much do they want it? If they say 10, well, does this mean they would sell their whole possessions to get it? I think that anywhere above 5 or 6 is okay because this means they would put themselves out for the outcome, hand over some hard-earned cash and would really like to bring about the change that brought them to me. Some people have health issues which, by making the change, may just disappear or no longer be a problem. This is even better for me as the hypnotherapist as it means a lot more to the client to get the outcome.

The other very important factor is to be 'at cause'. Putting it simply, it means that whatever the problem is, the client must, to some degree, take responsibility. This does not mean that the problem is their fault necessarily, but that they take responsibility for the outcome. If you believe that, no matter what, there is a way out of, around or over the problem, it can be solved. You see, the problem is yours; you need to own it.

I am sure I speak for most people, that it is so much easier to blame the problem on someone, or something, else. 'It was too hard because …' 'I can't do it because …' etc. What you need to understand is that there can be no blame, only solutions. Yes, the situation you find yourself in may seem an impossible one, but given time and energy there surely is a way out.

I will give you an example to help you understand more clearly the concept. Is it your fault if you get abused by someone you love? The answer is no, but it is your responsibility. Now, please don't get offended when I say this, as there is reason for it. It is not your fault but it is your responsibility to remove yourself from this abusive situation. If that person swears they love you, then that may be so in their model of the world, but not in most people's. They may have been abused by their own parents and then have trapped in their unconscious mind that abuse is love.

Most of us, of course, would not agree with this concept because our model of the world would be that understanding, caress and kindness is love. The responsibility to change is with both the person who is being abused and the abuser. It can be done, but only if both agree to seek the help needed to rescue this relationship.

Another example is when someone says they are addicted to something. Some addictions are true addictions, such as with many hard drugs because they make changes to our body. Once that drug is no longer there the body goes into withdrawal. Withdrawal from drugs can be done with hypnosis. However, much has to be known about the withdrawal and the symptoms and effects on the mind and body during withdrawal.

With food and cigarettes, however, the craving is more with the mind rather than cravings of withdrawal. Why else are some people able to give up without a problem with hypnotherapy, or if they are told that they have a life-threatening illness? Yes, they may have 'cravings' during withdrawal, but often these are due to the client thinking that they are 'missing out' on something rather than signs of bodily withdrawal. No one wants to think that they are losing something. Therefore, convincing them that, instead, they are gaining so much more or filling the void with something else is much more palatable.

Let's get back on track now. Being 'at cause' means taking responsibility. Remember, before you say, 'I can't', first think how you can. Don't forget that it is much easier to blame than to take the blame, and much easier to walk away than to work out how to right the wrong and stay.

In the next chapters I will share with you a little about how hypnotherapy can work and how the magic happens.

Chapter 3
Frequently Asked Questions

I find that people mainly ask the same questions when they are considering hypnotherapy. If I can answer them here and now, then I feel that the decision of whether or not to try hypnotherapy should be easier. So, here goes.

What is hypnotherapy?

Hypnotherapy is a very old method of helping people to change their mind about a problem, or to help with an illness or a 'dis ease'. I say 'dis ease' because it is believed, in some circles, that a disease occurs when the body is not at ease with what is happening. It is uneasy and, therefore, allows illness to occur. Hypnosis or hypnotherapy has been documented as far back as 1500 and has gone in and out of fashion. Some of those ancient techniques are still being used today in one way or another.

Hypnotherapy is a method of deep relaxation (or trance) – a state in which the subconscious mind can be accessed completely and told that it wants to listen and take on what is said as it is important for the client's well-being.

The method I use is the Krasner method, developed in 1982 by A. M. Krasner, but similar techniques were used as far back as 1500. This deep relaxation is achieved by getting the client to relax each part of their body, breathing deeply and taking them to a place (in their subconscious) where they feel not only relaxed but safe and peaceful. This technique is called the 'induction'. It is good at this time to also use some VACOG. This is short for Visual, Auditory, Kinaesthetic, Olfactory and Gustatory stimuli to reinforce the visualisation of the induction.

What I mean by this is that I may ask you to imagine yourself in a forest or garden. To reinforce that image, I will ask you to smell the scent of flowers, notice the colours and feel the breeze or the sun on your face. Although these are all in your mind, they make you feel that you really are there. It is almost like being inside a movie and is all done to help the relaxation happen. This will help to calm the subconscious mind as well as calm the body. It is like getting the attention of an overactive child.

Normally, when not relaxed, the subconscious mind takes in over 150 pieces of information per second, including visual, auditory, kinaesthetic and things remembered. That is an awful lot of information, most of which is deleted as not necessary, but nonetheless is taken in.

Hypnosis quietens the mind and helps it to take in the important things, some of which is information that is known by the conscious mind — for example, that the chemicals contained in cigarettes are dangerous to your health. You may say that everyone knows this, and you would be right. However, what the subconscious mind may have taken in is 'My father smoked for 40 years and died of a heart attack. His death was not lung related; therefore, it is okay to smoke.'

Of course, smoking probably did still kill their father, as it hardens the arteries and can cause a heart attack. The fact that he also died at the age of 60 means that he cut his lifespan by approximately 25 years by doing so. You see, we tell ourselves many little lies to make it seem that what we are doing is okay when, in fact, it really isn't.

Because the subconscious mind is like a captive audience, we can delete those lies and replace them with what is needed to resolve our problem. The hypnotist may tell stories, called metaphors, as the subconscious loves stories that it can decipher. These stories need not even make sense in the real world and it really doesn't matter as long as the moral of the story does.

For instance, I tell smokers who hate the smell of smoke a story about a skunk that smelled so bad that even his friends, who were all skunks, couldn't stand the smell. His name is Stinky and his story of how he lost his terrible smell helps those who have a problem with how they smell of cigarette smoke. Some clients may not worry about this and, therefore, this story may not make that impact, so I would leave it out and choose something else that does.

Hypnosis, or trance, is only part of the whole thing, though, and the therapy side – making sure that the client is in a positive state, telling them how good they will feel, how proud of themselves they will be, etc. – is a much larger part. Making people feel good about their decision to change and how good they will feel as a result is paramount in helping with this change.

As therapists, we are never here to judge. A client may tell me that they have taken drugs, been in a deep depression, split from a partner, or whatever the problem may be, but none of this matters. The only thing that matters is getting the result. It doesn't matter how I feel about the subject; all I care about is the right outcome. When that person leaves my office feeling relaxed and ready to take on the world, it is the best feeling in the whole world. Believe me, it can't get any better than that for both therapist and client!

Is hypnotherapy mind control?

Not at all. You can wake up from the hypnosis any time you want. If the therapist says something that may compromise your beliefs, say religiously, either your unconscious mind will simply delete it or you will just wake up. You will only take on what you like.

If I said that your spirit had a previous life and you just didn't believe in spirits, then you would delete that piece of information and move on. It would not normally knock out the rest of the session, but it could if it was something that really did not sit well with you. Similarly, if I said go and jump off a high building, would you? No, of course not because your conscious mind wouldn't let you, as it knows that this is a stupid and dangerous thing to do.

I explain this concept as the conscious and the unconscious minds being like the captain and the crew of a ship; they both have to work together or the ship goes nowhere. If I tell your unconscious mind to do something that the conscious mind is opposed to, it just will not happen. It is you who has come with the problem and you who wants the change to happen, so I am just the person who makes that happen.

What does it feel like to be hypnotised?

It is very much like the time before sleep, or when you are watching a movie and start to drop off whilst doing so. You feel very relaxed but are still able to hear sounds and, if asked to, can respond by either words or nodding of the head. Often you will be asked to nod your head in agreement with a statement. This means that you agree with what is being asked and it is not as disruptive to the relaxation as speaking.

Saying that, I did have a client once who forgot to turn off his telephone. It rang whilst he was deeply under hypnosis, and he looked at it, turned it off and went straight back into the state he'd been in. The outcome was still as good as if there were no interruption. Everyone is almost surprised when they come out of hypnosis as to how wonderful and relaxed they feel upon waking.

How will I know that it has worked?

Many people don't know at first if the hypnotherapy has worked. Mostly it seems to just creep up on you. You think about the problem differently or you start doing things which surprise you.

I can give you an example. A client of mine wanted to give up sweet things, especially chocolate. She said she had never walked down the chocolate aisle of the supermarket without buying some sort of chocolate or, at least, lollies. When she was on a diet she would study each packet to see which ones were the least calorific. She still could not walk away without something. We exchanged lollies for fruits. She called me after our session as she had walked into the supermarket after leaving me and had arrived home and opened the bag only to find blueberries. She couldn't even remember buying them – just that she had seen them on special. She had no recollection of walking even as far as the lolly aisle. 'Great work,' I told her. 'Carry on.'

It is obvious that something had happened. Exactly what, we cannot say and with some people it just happens on the spot. They walk out without even remembering what problem brought them to me as it has already disappeared from their mind. With some people, however, it may take a couple of weeks to kick in. It may be, in this instance, that they will not even credit the hypnotherapy with being the reason for the change. It does, though, seem funny that they weren't able to accomplish the change without help prior to the hypnosis. That is fine, as long as the result has been reached and the client got the outcome they wanted.

What is the cost?

I try to make the sessions so that most people can afford them. I know this may seem crazy, because how can you put a price on things like your mental or physical health?

I once had someone tell me that $200 was something she just couldn't justify paying to give up alcohol. I didn't argue with her, but it did make me wonder if she thought that the $20-

$30 dollars a day that she spent on alcohol was well spent? How much did she think it would cost for all the hospitalisation she would need in the future, and could she put a cost on the family and friends that she had lost because of her over indulgence?

It is funny how we often see money. Is the money we spend spent well? Will it save us in the long run, and is our health really so under-valued? Those are not questions for me to ask unless a person has come to me for advice, guidance and to quit their behaviour.

If so, then those are some very tough questions that I would be putting forward for my client to think about and to try and put into perspective.

All I can say is, ask yourself, 'Is this problem enough for me to spend x amount of dollars trying to rid myself of?' 'If this was an appointment to see a specialist, would I do it?' If it was, say, an MRI to show the damage already done, would you? This $$xxx$ could potentially save your life, or at least make your life a whole lot better. You have to weigh up the cost vs the savings and ask, 'What is the investment … and do I think I will get a good return on that investment?'

Will I immediately feel different?

Good question. It may be that when you come out of trance you will immediately feel different. Some clients have felt differently about the problem that brought them to me. It can be a little odd, but most often people will work their way into the change. A bit like gaining momentum, they start out by thinking differently and then find that their mind is convinced that it does not want to do a particular behaviour anymore.

I once treated someone who said she had great trouble when talking to, or seeing, her mother. They just did not see eye to eye, and it made her upset every time her mother was on the telephone or came to the house and she just didn't want that to happen, because deep down she loved her mother. Imagine how delighted she was when I saw her next after her mother had telephoned her only hours after the hypnosis. Her mother said something that would normally have started an argument but all the client said was, 'That's okay, Mum. You have your opinion and I have mine, but that's okay, isn't it?'

She said her mother was so taken aback that she stopped shouting and put the phone down. It was even funnier, a couple of days later her mother visited and said, 'You know, there is something different about you. I like it!'

There was nothing more said, but they got on so much better from then on. No more fighting and bickering. My client had no idea where that calmness came from; it just happened.

You will see from my client profiles in the chapters 'Short and Sweet' and 'OMG' that it may or may not happen instantaneously. Do not be put off if it takes a week or two to kick in. Once it does, you will know. Believe me, things start to change and when they do, look out world!

What happens if I can't wake up at the end?

That just isn't a thing. You may be reluctant to come back to the room, and by this I mean it may take a second or two and you might be a little disorientated, but really, that is all. You may find that you are so relaxed you need a minute or two to come round, but once you do you will feel fantastic, not only because you have been so relaxed, but also because, as I have already said, hypnotherapy works with the positive. You will have been given a new slant on your problem and been given positive words, phrases and metaphors that give you a great feeling when returning to the room. The reaction that I usually get is, 'Wow, that was fantastic!'

That is why included with this book is a session for relaxation. You can download it from my website, so you will be able to listen to it any time you like. It doesn't matter that it isn't made with only you in mind, because relaxation is great at any time, for anyone. I hope you will love it as much as I have loved creating it!

I hope these 7 questions have helped you to think more about hypnosis in general, or to ask yourself, 'Could hypnotherapy be for me?'

Chapter 4
Is hypnotherapy magic or magical?

To some people whom I have treated, the way that hypnotherapy works can seem like magic. They have a problem that they really want addressed, and may even need to remove from their lives. For them it seems simple: they come in, we talk, I hypnotise them, problem solved. I can tell you that from my side there is much more to it, of course, or otherwise people would be able to make that change themselves. If they go away thinking that it is magic, that is fine, as long as the desired outcome is obtained.

To me, hypnotherapy is definitely magical, though. I cannot tell you how good it feels when someone hugs me and walks away from my room a changed person. Getting them the result that they want is paramount to my work. I am not there to judge if the thing they come to change is their biggest issue, either. You see, it is their problem and their solution. It is important for me to understand that not everyone wants to tackle the hard stuff, but I let them know that at any time if they want or need to tackle other problems I will be right there.

I once had a client who wanted to get over a phobia of flying. She had been to see another therapist who wanted to treat some underlying problems. The client was not satisfied bringing up her unhappy past. Fair enough – not everyone wants or needs to go back there and sort it out. We sorted out the phobia and she walked away. I told her that if ever she wanted to go and sort the past out, I would be happy to help.

As yet, she hasn't been back, and that is completely her call. I hope she will come back as much of our past can leave an impression on our future and it is for this reason that I always try to be available, even if it means coming to the office late at night or on a Sunday or public holiday, etc. Everyone is important and if that problem is important to them, then it is to me!

I want to talk a little about how the magic happens and the behind the scenes stuff. When looking at how to resolve problems and what is necessary to change, it is important to look at the six basic human needs. These human needs are very important to know when deciding on a pathway to success, and to solving a client's problem.

These are the six human needs:

- Certainty
- Uncertainty
- Significance
- Connection
- Growth
- Contribution

I am going to try and help you to understand more by giving an example. Let us take an alcohol-dependent person to show their human needs and how they are met by consuming alcohol and how they can change this destructive behaviour.

Certainty

We all like to be certain of things. We like the security it gives us and we feel safe if we know how things are going to be. For instance, if you drink a bottle of vodka you will feel drunk. If someone knows this, and then this feels good, why would they change it? The reason why most people want to change this habit is because they feel that they cannot function well without it. The fact that their health suffers (especially their liver) and also their relationships, etc. does not seem to be seen as a problem. However, the 'not being able to function without it' is. If they are wanting to change that, then where is that certainty? It has gone!

The way you make this magic work is by telling them that the certainty is from knowing that without the alcohol they will certainly improve their health and be able to function much better as they will have a clearer mind and, with time, will gain back trust and so relationships with others will improve, and the relationship with themselves, too. They will feel more in control, have self-respect (something that has possibly been missing for some time) and self-belief.

Uncertainty

Yes, believe it or not, the human need of uncertainty is there, too. We all like that little flutter in the stomach when we meet uncertainty. We like to feel that we are not totally in control. That is why when we undertake something new it sets off those butterflies. The same with the alcohol problem: What if they have to sneak the bottle in — will it be seen? Can they get away without someone noticing? How drunk can they really get? What if they try two bottles — what will the outcome be?

All those things lead to uncertainty and wondering what the outcome will be. If we put a different slant on uncertainty to help them overcome their problem, we may say, 'How will the person feel if they don't have that alcohol but instead do something different that is exciting? What if they try talking to people sober instead of drunk? Might people be more responsive as they are now coherent and speak sensibly? How much money could they save and where could that money take them?' Those things that make them uncertain in a good way outweigh all the uncertainties of the alcohol for sure, and it is with the positive uncertainties that the magic can happen.

Significance

Many people see significance from people caring for themselves, and that can even be when someone is actually causing them harm. As long as they are getting attention then they are significant. Many people who drink do not care about themselves too much — they have lost their own respect, but to the people who love them it is devastating. Those people, though, often tend to try and influence the alcohol-affected person by caring for them – giving them food, washing their clothes, encouraging them to 'do the right thing'.

What the unconscious mind may think, however, is, 'If I give up drinking then I have to care for myself. If I do care for myself then will everyone just forget me? I may have to get a job, and with no alcohol on board that would be a scary thing to do.' (An alcoholic may not have worked for a long time, and getting a job in itself would be very intimidating.) Much has to change in the conscious mind of an alcoholic to change their unconscious mind. It can be done, though, I assure you. When it comes to significance, however, if the person already has a job or still has a friend or family who love them, then this part is made one hundred times easier.

Connection

This is similar to 'significance', whereby the alcoholic loses touch with reality. They lose touch with people and become more and more withdrawn, spending much of their time alone. This lack of connection is not only with friends and family, but with the world and also themselves, more often than not. They feel isolated and alone.

It is very important for them to try and reconnect with at least one true friend, or connect with someone who does not know too much about their past, allowing them to become their true self again, instead of the alcohol-affected person. This, in turn, will connect them to the person they were before the alcohol took their self-worth, self-respect and self-confidence. Once they have made a connection with themselves, at least one other person (and maybe family, depending their circumstances as it is harder to get back trust and respect from family) then it is time to reconnect with the outside world. The best thing to do is some charity work, especially with the under-privileged. No more sitting alone with nothing to do, as this just feeds that disconnection.

Growth

Everyone needs to grow, just like every living thing. This growth can be achieved in many ways. By this I mean by studying something, or growing something themselves (produce to be shared is even better) because nothing can beat eating something from your own garden or planter. It is fresh with no pesticides or additives and is clean and so good for your body. An alcoholic could do something that will spiritually grow them such as a course in something holistic. They should talk about their problem and get it out because, as they say, 'a problem shared is a problem halved'.

The person should try to understand how they got to this point. What strategies can they use to change so that they can love themselves and love life? If they have done some things in the past that are haunting them, they can just decide that it can't be changed but they can change the future. They can say sorry to those whom they have hurt, and really mean it, but then move on. The things that were done cannot be undone, but it is not time to dwell on those. Let them go.

Contribution

This isn't written now just for the person with the problem but for all of us. It is so important to give back whenever and wherever you can. If you can afford time and not money, then donate your time. Time is always better than money, of course, as the connection is also important to them.

Does a local library need help, or a retirement home? Try to find a charity that hits a chord with you – there are so many out there. Local charities can be wonderful as they may even have collectors at local events that you can go to, to increase your connection as well as contribution. It is so important that a person feels that they are contributing to society, as an alcohol-dependent person may think that they are not seen to be caring about anything other than where their next bottle of alcohol is coming from. This contribution increases their self-worth and respect from those around them.

Applying the human needs to hypnotherapy

When preparing a session, it is important to not only know a little about the client but also to know how best to help their subconscious mind take on the change needed. Keeping in mind the above human needs, it is important to know the client's beliefs around the change needing to take place. It is a case of creating the mindset that the change is possible.

As I have said in a previous chapter, you just need to believe that change can happen and it will. If you believe that alcohol does not harm your body, then I have to have some valid proof that it does. Everyone knows this to be true; however, the person with an alcohol problem may have told themselves that they are different and that they will not sustain harm or illness from over-consumption of alcohol. That, of course, is a lie in the majority of cases. They may have seen a movie in which the hero has a problem with alcohol and still does miraculous things. This is not reality, though, is it?

In my profession as a nurse, I have seen many patients ruin their lives through consuming too much alcohol, and the prognosis is grim. If you decide to give up whilst young, however, then the chances are that you will live a full and active life. If not, get ready for a rough road ahead! The unconscious mind, though, loves the truth and because hypnotherapy works on giving the mind all the positives rather than the negatives, then it likes what it hears.

Yes, hypnotherapy works on trying to convince the subconscious in a positive way. In this way, the problem can be called just that – 'the problem' – so that there is no labelling, for example alcoholic, depressed person, etc. These can all be talked about as 'the problem'. The client will know what this means to them. This also means that if there is a solution to every problem, then the problem can be solved.

In a hypnotherapy session, instead of talking

about isolation, we talk about how it feels to be happy and loved, turning away from the word and feeling of isolation. If the client is finding it hard to imagine how it feels to be happy, then you can take them back to a time when they were happy in the past. Most people can find a time, a specific time, when they were happy. Once they find that time, you can tell them that they can find that feeling again. Changing their state of mind helps greatly, so they can see that the happiness is still an option for them. It may not be easy to feel that happiness 24/7, but they can still feel how it is to be happy.

I know I have talked mainly about alcohol as an example but it works the same for anything we treat, really. When you identify the problem and the client is at cause for the problem, then it is only coming up with a solution that is involved.

A client once said that no one ever told them that their depression could go away. When they saw a psychologist, they discussed how their depression was going and how they were able to 'manage' it but never talked about the possibility that if the problem that caused the depression went away, then so, too, would the depression.

The label of depression is a very heavy burden to carry because not only is mental illness still taboo, but it is hard to distinguish between a depression caused by an event, or one that is intrinsic and seems to happen for no apparent reason. I do not want to touch too much on the subject of mental health, but it just may be that if you have a mental condition it is possible that you can live without it. If I were living with a big black cloud covering my whole being I would do anything to try and lift it, blow it away, or put a big bright light above my head to outshine it. Yes, there are many solutions to one problem!

I hope I have given you food for thought – a bright light at the end of a tunnel – so that you can, if necessary, find hypnotherapy to be the answer to your specific problem. It doesn't matter how big or small, how strange or 'normal' the problem is, if it is a problem for you, then you just might be able to find a solution. The next chapter is evidence! They say that the proof is in the pudding (where did that saying come from?) – people believe what they see and hear.

This is the reason why I have written this book. If hypnotherapy can work for the people in these stories, then why not for you? I wanted to include some smaller problems, but problems nonetheless. Then I wanted to have a couple of 'OMG' stories because I know you will be saying things like WTF! Enjoy!

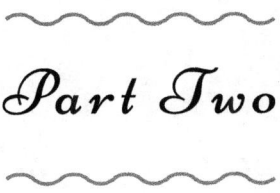

Chapter 5
Short and Sweet

This chapter is all about other people's stories. This is quite simply normal, everyday people like you and me who have had transformations with the help of hypnotherapy. They wanted to change something in their lives and decided to give hypnosis a try and, in doing so, have transformed their lives in some way. This may seem small to those of us who do not have the problem, but to them it may mean spending many more years with their loved ones, having more money in their pockets or being able to study more effectively.

I want everyone to see that just a little shift in one direction can have a snowball effect throughout their whole lives. The people in this book were either clients of mine, friends, family, or from my hypnosis family (people who have been trained by Shane and Jess who have become like family). Each one of them has given their story freely and I thank every one of them. I have changed the names of some of these clients in order to maintain their privacy. I hope you enjoy their stories and get some hope for your own transformation.

Anne-Marie's story

Profile: Nurse, aged mid-40s, married with three children

I had been working with Benetta for a few years – we worked on the Oncology ward together. I knew that she had just finished a course in hypnotherapy and was looking for volunteers to try it out. I trusted Benetta and we had a good relationship, so it was quite easy to volunteer. I wasn't scared of trying it out as I knew she would never let anything bad happen to me.

We arranged for me to come to her house one day. She asked me what I would like to change or if there was anything giving me trouble. At first, I couldn't really think of anything in particular; however, I had always had a thing for lollies. It didn't matter what they were – chocolate was my favourite – but if it wasn't there, anything would do. It wasn't just one or two, it was handfuls at a time. I mean, it was a real problem for me to say no!

Benetta was very professional in her approach and asked me if I had a connection with lollies. 'What does she mean,' I thought, 'a connection?' I thought about it for a while, and then something did occur to me. My grandmother and my father always had a large jar of lollies in their home, as I had always had in mine.

Really? Could this be the connection Benetta was talking about? We went on to discuss a little about that connection and she asked, 'Could you make a better connection with your grandmother and father than eating all those bad things?' 'Well,' I said, 'maybe that I look like them, or that people have always said I have the same personality – happy and love to help people.' 'Great,' she said. 'Do you feel happier with that connection rather than the one you had?' I actually did. It was amazing to feel that connection to my family members again, as both of them had passed away some time before.

Benetta said it was really easy to hypnotise me, even though I had never done it before. I just felt so relaxed and at ease. It was a great feeling, sort of like being in that half-awake and half-asleep phase. It was so good; my body felt heavy and I just didn't want to move. She said I was hypnotised for about 40 minutes but it seemed like only a couple of minutes. I really didn't want to wake up afterwards as I was so comfortable. I can't remember exactly what she said to wake me up, but when I woke up I felt so light, and I felt relieved in a funny way. When I woke up, I really wasn't sure if the hypnosis had worked. I wasn't expecting it to, to be honest; I just did it to help out.

It wasn't long before I was tested. I went home and the lolly jar was there. I would normally just hoe in and not think about it until afterwards. I was amazed that I really didn't know if I wanted the lollies or not. It was a bit of a strange feeling, as if I was second-guessing myself.

I had another funny thing start to happen: when chocolates were brought out at work (as always happens) I wouldn't have one, but after they were finished I would feel as if I had missed out on something. That feeling went on for a couple of weeks – a sort of twilight zone of not having any sweet things and then wondering if I was missing out. I could almost taste them without having any. It was most peculiar! I hadn't told anyone that I had the hypnosis because I felt people wouldn't be understanding and would test me. I really didn't want testing, even though I was sort of testing myself all the time.

In a few weeks, however, it was so apparent to everyone as I hadn't had any sweets, chocolates, cakes, etc. at all. I no longer wanted them and I could just walk away and not feel that I was missing out on anything. The feeling of not wanting them at all just gets stronger and stronger, even to the extent of feeling quite sick when thinking about having one. One day, I stupidly put a Tic Tac in my mouth without thinking and had to spit it straight out as it was just too sweet to stand.

It's been a year now and I feel an even stronger connection to my grandmother and father now. I loved them both dearly. I really feel so much better for not eating those sweet things. I used to feel guilty for eating them as I knew how bad it was for me, but now I am guilt-free and sweets-free!

***

It was a pleasure doing the hypnosis for Anne-Marie. She was a great subject for me to practise on as it gave me confidence to continue and to treat people as a practitioner. I wanted to include her in my 'Short and Sweet' section as her story shows that even small changes can mean a great deal to people. Anne-Marie is not overweight but, still, things like sugar can be very harmful, especially in large doses. In this instance, she may have saved herself getting diabetes.

I also wanted to showcase that even if a client is a friend, if they have trust in you, then it really doesn't matter if they are sceptical about the outcome; it can still work. Also, I wanted to show that sometimes the mind takes a while to deal with the whole process. It's like the mind is weighing up the pros and cons and then comes to a decision that is the right one, the one that the client chose. The feeling becomes stronger and stronger as time goes on. I think it was very brave and wonderful that Anne-Marie took a chance on me.

Bethan's story

Profile: University student, aged 23, and my daughter

My mum and I are really close and when she decided to go and see what hypnotherapy was all about she took me along. It was great to learn something new, and I really liked it. It seemed like a great way to get people to sort out their problems, give up things that were bad for them, or even just to relax.

One of the most memorable hypnosis sessions for me was regarding getting a job that I was being interviewed for. I had wanted to work in retail (a part-time job whilst at university) instead of hospitality. I hadn't done any retail work, but all of a sudden I got an interview (this had never happened to me for a retail job before) and I was shocked at even getting an interview for this position. I always got nervous before interviews anyway and ended up saying stupid things, so I asked Mum to do some hypnosis.

I was getting ready and, for some reason, didn't get the awful butterflies in my stomach that I usually got when going for an interview. I just knew I was going to get the job! (Looking back on it, I'm not sure what would have happened if I didn't get it.) I just remember walking in and being confident. The girl interviewing me even threw me a blind-sided question: 'Who is your favourite super hero?' OMG, I didn't do super heroes – that was my brother's field of expertise! 'Sailor Moon' came out of my mouth before I could even think. She smiled. 'I love Sailor Moon,' she said.

After we talked for a bit, the interviewer said, 'I will let you know.' Deflated, I walked away, feeling that maybe I blew it. Then the phone rang; they wanted me. I hadn't even left the building. There have been many more times that I have used hypnosis and I am sure it has not been the last!

I have included Bethan's story to highlight the fact that it doesn't matter whether the client is family, friend or a stranger; if the issue at hand is something important to that person, hypnotherapy can work.

Emily's story

Profile: Therapist, aged mid-30s, married with two children in late teens

I had been battling an addiction with wine for years. I am a wife and a mother of two and every day I would drink a glass of wine. I felt that was okay, but then that glass crept to two and then to a half a bottle and then to a bottle. You would probably call me a high functioning alcoholic. I never let it come in the way of my home life or working life … or so I thought.

Then I started to makes excuses to get home early so that I could start drinking. I would forget conversations I had with my family and I would repeat myself. I was unmotivated and becoming overweight, lazy and fuzzy in the head. I would wake up every day with a hangover. I was only wanting wine, not beer or spirits – I could go without those altogether as they didn't interest me.

I would go without alcohol at all sometimes, but then something would happen and it would consume me. It would take over and I would drink, no matter what. I didn't have the excuse that it was because I was sad, because I would drink if I was happy or sad, with friends or by myself; I had no excuses.

What I did do, though, was surround myself with other wine drinkers so that I didn't look so bad – you see, my husband doesn't drink! That meant I would sit alone at home and I distanced myself from my husband so that he didn't see what I was doing. Our relationship was suffering, and our sex life too. I really did not want this to happen as I really love him very much. My kids, too – what sort of role model was I as they were getting toward the age of going out, partying and drinking themselves?

I tried a lot of things to stop. More than anything, I wanted the ability to stop! I wanted to stop thinking about wine and start thinking about a solution. I just wanted it to go away.

I decided to turn to hypnotherapy. After just one hour-long session my addiction was gone. I could not believe it at first; I couldn't believe how easy it was. I have been around wine since my hypnotherapy session and friends have been drinking, but I just don't want it. Since the hypnotherapy, I have lost weight and am more motivated. I am closer than ever to my husband and children, and am really enjoying the high energy levels that I am experiencing. It has been fantastic, and I am looking to do some more hypnotherapy to accelerate learning and to process information more quickly.

***

It was good that Emily was open and really truthful about her problem. It takes a lot of courage to be that way and to tell someone else those things, but if a great outcome is going to be achieved it really is necessary, because it means the client is coming clean with themselves. It is not my place to be judgemental; however, the client needs to recognise the facts within themselves.

Emily told me that this wine drinking did have a starting point that was to do with coping with an abusive relationship. The relationship had long been over, but her relationship with wine really wasn't. It was easy to distance her from the wine and to replace it with a great alternative, something healthy and appealing (it happened to be sparkling mineral water with ice and lime or lemon.) I enticed her to like it even more with the sight, sound and taste of it.

I distanced her from the wine by calling it nasty names like 'parasite' and 'demon', so that she would associate it with something nasty and undesirable. The fact of thinking about it was replaced by thinking only of the connection with her husband and children, combined with feelings of self-worth, self-belief and wellbeing. Thrown in was the feeling of being healthier, the reduction of weight and her healthy liver. The job was complete. If the wine ever does rear its ugly head she knows that help is at hand ... but I doubt it will.

Linda's story

Profile: Aged care co-ordinator, aged mid-50s, divorced mother of three adult children and grandmother of one

I came to see Benetta as I was having trouble sleeping. It was getting so bad that I would wake several times a night and it felt as if I had no sleep at all. I had some problems at the time, and they would just keep going around and around in my head. I told myself to just go back to sleep and tried several other things that people had told me to try, but nothing worked. I was getting more and more tired and couldn't function anymore. It was getting hard to even go to work as I was so depleted in energy. I wasn't sure that I really believed in hypnotherapy, but by this time I was willing to give anything a try to feel better.

While I was under hypnosis, my mind kept thinking, 'This isn't working. I don't think I can be hypnotised.' Then, all of a sudden, those thoughts disappeared and I felt calm – somehow relaxed, but not intentionally. It just happened. When I spoke to Benetta afterwards and she asked me how I'd felt, I really wasn't sure. All I knew was that I felt somehow lighter; I don't know why, but I just did.

That night I was all ready to put it to the test. I didn't really sleep any better. I was a bit disappointed really, as I did want it to work, but it didn't. For a few nights afterwards I did the same, and still nothing happened. Finally, I stopped thinking about it, and possibly one or two weeks later I realised that I had been sleeping through the night, feeling better, and I had more energy. I cannot really remember when I started sleeping through. It was weird, as if I had forgotten to think about it and it just happened. It has been some 8 months since then, and I never think about it. I just go to bed and, believe me, I have had some big problems going on since that time, but they just don't keep me awake anymore!

***

This was an easy fix, really, as all that was necessary was to tell Linda's unconscious mind that nothing can be fixed whilst sleeping. Sleeping is so that your body and mind can function successfully. It is important for that to happen – otherwise, she would burn out and not be of any help to anyone in that state. If she did sleep, however, her job to help the person whom she was worrying about would be much easier. Day time is for sorting problems and worrying; night time is for sleeping. (The worrying was at least warranted. Day time worrying is only okay if you should be worried.)

Georgina's story

Profile: Shop owner, aged mid-50s, divorced with three adult children

I heard about Benetta from my friend Linda. Linda had been successful in sleeping so well since seeing Benetta and so I thought I would see if she could help me. I was really stressed, mainly at work. I worked with my brother and my sister; we owned a shop. There was a lot going on between us all. I kept thinking back to when we were young and how well we all got on. It was upsetting and I hated the way we all weren't getting along. I am the eldest and it was always my job to look after everyone and I didn't like how things were. I just wanted to feel better and less stressed about everything.

Benetta and I had a long chat and even before the hypnosis I started to feel better about things. During the hypnosis, I just remember feeling so relaxed and don't remember much about what was said, but when I woke up I felt so much better. I felt that I could cope a lot better. The things that had really worried me just didn't anymore. I thought I could let those things go. I knew that much of what was happening wasn't down to me, so I couldn't change these things, but what I could do was just let them go. It was strange how only my mindset changed – nothing else, as I had to continue to work there, for the time being; I had to work with the people who had caused me to feel stressed. The only thing that changed was my attitude to those problems. It was great! I felt free!

***

Sometimes it just isn't feasible to tell a person to leave. People aren't always in a position to leave a job, partner or whatever the problem is. However, something has to change. If you are feeling overwhelmed by something and if you want the situation to change, change *must* occur. If nothing changes, then change cannot occur! It was apparent that Georgina had to stay in the job, for the short term at least, and work with her siblings. So if the change cannot come from either her leaving, or them leaving, then what had to change was the way in which she saw the problem.

This is not always easy, but I have found that if you even leave people with those few words, 'Nothing changes if nothing changes', it brings about a change, if change is what they need or desire. It is made even easier by bringing in that wondrous thing called 'Cause and Effect' or, really, it could be called, 'No more Excuses!' I know we, as humans, love to play that game of blame.

Georgina came back to see me, thankfully not about her first problem but for something else completely. Here is what she said:

I came back to see Benetta as my siblings and I decided to sell the shop and go our separate ways. It was time to take a break as I had been working non-stop at the shop, and when it is your own business it is hard to take a proper break. My sister, sister-in-law and I decided to go back to the 'old country' (Greece) and then to travel around Europe. We had made all the arrangements and then, for some strange reason, I started panicking. I mean, I didn't even know why, but this was a real feeling of dread, almost to a point of cancelling completely.

I had this knot in my stomach that wouldn't go away and I was sick about it. I needed help! I went to Benetta and again we talked a little about my situation and started to realise that this was stupid. I already really knew this, but I couldn't stop how I felt. She gathered some details about the holiday such as where we were going and why. While I was under hypnosis, she took me to some of those places that I had been to and the happiness I felt there. It was as if I really was there. It was a fantastic feeling!

After the session, I just wanted to go … like, that very minute. I was ready and feeling fantastic. I went on that holiday and I was calm, even when the flight was delayed. I didn't care at all and I even calmed the others down. The holiday was the best thing ever. I enjoyed every single moment of it and I just want to go again.

***

This was also so easy to deal with, especially as Georgina had done so well after the first session she'd had. It is much easier once hypnosis has been performed before because not only is the client prepared for how it feels to be hypnotised, but they also have faith in the practitioner. Plain sailing ahead! I just told Georgina that this was her time, and she would have the time of her life! There was a bit more to it, but really it was easy for me and easy for her, too.

Scott's story

Profile: Builder, aged late 50s, married with two children

I wanted and needed to give up smoking. I had gotten to the stage where I just didn't want to do that anymore. I am a footy coach and wanted to be a role model for those boys. I knew that they knew that I smoked, as they would see me outside smoking at training. I also knew that I smelled bad; the smoky smell following me around was awful. My wife doesn't smoke so it should have been easy for me to do this on my own but whenever I tried, I couldn't do it.

I would stop for a day or two, but then I always went back to it. I felt bad for not being able to do it alone, but I thought 'Let's give it a go.' I really wasn't sure that hypnotherapy would work, though. What did I really have to lose? Okay, I could lose some money if it didn't work, but what if it did?

I was pretty sceptical when I walked in, but after my first session in which Benetta talked about many aspects about smoking and then took some personal details about me so that she could make the hypnosis as personal as possible, I felt much more at ease and started to believe that it could happen. I felt excited instead of scared! I couldn't wait for the next day so that I could complete the session.

I was told to go home and collect up anything that reminded me of smoking. That was everything in my home, car and work. I was asked to bring it all to Benetta's room the next day. This gave me all night to deliberate on my decision to give up.

The next day, I buried my Mum and, under normal circumstances, the stress of that event would have made me change my mind, but on that day I just seemed even more convinced that this was the right decision.

By the time I arrived at Benetta's room I was ready. It was a little weird, that feeling of wanting to give up so much now, but I was totally ready. I threw the bag with the cigarettes, lighter, ash tray, etc. into the bin and said my final good-bye. In approximately 40 minutes, I was going to not only become an ex-smoker but a non-smoker. This label was better for me because I was told that it then completely cut me off from smoking. You see, an ex-smoker might have the feeling that they need just one more, or envy those smoking. As a non-smoker, I wouldn't even think about smoking because someone who does not smoke never thinks about smoking.

Benetta had me sit in a very soft and comfortable chair. She told me that it was okay if my mind seemed to wander because that was my conscious mind, but that it was the unconscious mind she needed to contact, and the more relaxed I was the easier it was to reach the unconscious mind.

As I sat, relaxing, I couldn't believe how easy it was to relax. I thought I would be tense and restless but, no, it was easy. I can't remember most of the things Benetta said at that time, but a couple of things did stick – the ones that were very personal to me. Looking back, I think that those things made a big impact. Before I knew it, it was time to wake up. The time seemed to pass so quickly, and when Benetta said it had been about 40 minutes, I just couldn't believe it!

Then the funniest thing happened. Benetta asked, 'How do you feel now about that old problem that brought you here today?' I recall trying to think of the problem, and I just couldn't. Even the thought of it had just disappeared. I really don't know how that would happen as I had smoked since being a teenager, so for 40 years.

I left the room and haven't touched a cigarette since! I don't think about them and have absolutely no desire to smoke. I have told all my friends about it and have given Benetta's name to them all. I don't really know how it worked; I just know it did, effortlessly. If you want to change from being a smoker to a non-smoker, I highly recommend hypnotherapy in order to do so.

***

Many hypnotherapists think of smoking cessation as either their 'bread and butter' type of hypnosis, or as a specialised type. I just think that it is fantastic to help someone who is, in reality, self-harming. As a nurse, I have seen many people have emphysema or lung cancer from smoking cigarettes. It is heart-breaking for not only the person who is sick but for their family. The guilt that the person feels, too, is enormous because they know that had they stopped smoking years ago they may well not be in this state.

I am happy to say, though, that I have had many young people see the light long before they have caused themselves lung damage. Well done to those people and also to people like Scott, who really wanted to be a good role model to the young people he coached.

Chapter 6
OMG

I have separated the stories into the two groups so that I can showcase how even problems of a physical nature or complex as quitting drugs can be done. Giving up drugs should not be done lightly, of course, and there are certain drugs that are known to have dangerous withdrawal symptoms, but with care this process can still be undertaken with hypnotherapy.

I was told by Jasmine (one of the clients whose story is in this chapter) that she had read somewhere that giving up smoking is akin to giving up heroin. Jasmine had needed to give up smoking cigarettes. She was having an operation and needed to give up, but she didn't necessarily want to give up just yet. She was probably looking for an excuse to feel withdrawal and uneasy with the decision being made, more or less, for her. I told her that if she could give up the lifestyle she was living and replace it with how her life was so far, then giving up smoking should also be easy. However, each problem is different, isn't it?

I cannot believe how many people will Google something and then blindly believe what they read. Please, everyone, do not believe everything you read. Gather some information if you like, but then decipher it for yourself. Also, it is important to not label yourself. What I mean by this is, 'I suffer from depression', or 'I am a smoker', an 'alcoholic', etc. It may be that it has been the case that you have suffered from a condition, but anything can change.

In fact, everything changes minute to minute, hour to hour, day to day. Maybe yesterday you drank too much alcohol. Does this make you an alcoholic? No. If someone has done this day in, day out for a year, does this? You may say yes. I would like that person, however, to identify themselves as someone who turns to alcohol to help them cope. If they had a better method of coping and then were able to see the alcohol as a toxic friend – someone who was now making them sick, or losing friendships, etc. – then maybe they would not need the alcohol instead of saying that they were a mess, couldn't hold down a relationship and saw themselves as addicted.

Anyway, it is time for you to read Jasmine and Susie's stories so that you, too, can make up your mind about them. I want to thank these people for coming forward and telling their stories in order to, perhaps, help others to see that nothing is impossible!

Jasmine's story

Profile: Unemployed (at time of first hypnotherapy session), aged 21, in a new relationship

I was absolutely messed up. I was sick and smoking bongs every day, and having glasses of wine every second day and this was just during the week! When the long-awaited weekend came, my girlfriends and I would plan and set up what I would call a platter of drugs – uppers, downers, it didn't matter. The more twisted we got the better. I had been addicted to marijuana for over four years prior to this, but this raised partying lasted itself for about a year.

It was all I thought about; I was totally obsessed with drugs. I was rude to my family, had the biggest ego, and thought I was the smartest girl in the world. Throughout this time, I turned psychotic and my anxiety was through the roof. I was admitted to the hospital with psychosomatic pain. I thought people were talking about me behind my back and I constantly had nightmares of murdering people. It was terrible, but my view was 'be on drugs or die'. Those were my only choices.

I was caught driving under the influence of drink in August 2015. My licence was suspended for seven months. Fed up with my mental state and my addictions, I knew I was either going to make the best of the seven months or let myself spiral down. I decided that I could not let the latter happen. I had to make a change. That chance came along when I heard from a friend whom Benetta had helped to give up gambling. I needed help, and I thought, 'What have I got to lose?' You see, I was at breaking point. Something had to change. I had to change.

After just one session with Benetta, I started to believe that I could change. I went home and had no cravings for marijuana. I didn't even feel that I needed to smoke or anything. It felt so good and as though a great weight had been lifted from my shoulders. I could survive without it!

On the weekend my girlfriends and I had rented a house to celebrate a friend's birthday, and I knew there would be a lot of drugs happening. It was really going to test me. I passed people their drinks, I bought drugs at a club for my friends, had numerous drugs in front of me and people smoking marijuana too, but none of it triggered any interest in me. It was strange, as if I had never taken them; they were completely alien to me. It was the strangest experience ever, and when I was offered some, it was like seeing concrete on a plate – it was of no interest whatsoever! It was just so easy to say no.

It has been over nine months now and I feel the same. I know that Benetta is only a phone call away with good advice, and hypnosis if I need it. In fact, I have just given up smoking with her help, too. I need that money to go on a holiday – something I am planning in the next few months. I might even take up sport again, which has been missing from my life for quite some time.

My life has meaning now. I am no longer the girl who walked into Benetta's office. I like myself, I am proud of who I am and the direction that my life is going in. I am working, studying, in a great relationship, and feeling free. My family have got their daughter/sister back, and it is a fantastic feeling to be a part of their lives once again.

***

When Jasmine came to me, I instantly liked her. She had just turned 21 and was in a short-term relationship. I could tell she was troubled by her behaviour and she told me outright that she 'hated' herself. She wanted desperately to give up drugs and to be clean of them. I said I would only help if she could stay clean and sober for the next two days, and to come back to me two days later.

We talked a little about detox and the symptoms she may or may not have. She said that she was staying with people and would alert them to the fact that she was going to not be taking any drugs or alcohol for the next two days and maybe, if the plan worked, for ever. This was the task I had given her to prove that she was genuine and committed.

She was up for the challenge. When she came back, she said that she was very proud of herself as she had not been clean and sober for two days straight for a long time. This was a great start and I agreed that we should start right away. She really had no signs of withdrawal at all, not even anxiety which she had experienced in the past. After her first hypnotherapy session had finished, Jasmine cried quite a lot. The release of all the emotions made her feel so much better. We continued to see each other a few times after that and it is so rewarding to see the Jasmine within become the Jasmine of today. Congratulations to her for making the change, and for agreeing to tell her story.

Susie's story

Profile: Unemployed (at time of hypnotherapy), aged 73, divorced with one daughter and two grandchildren

Susie lives alone now but has a loving family of one daughter and two grandchildren. She had a strict Catholic upbringing but started learning alternative therapies when in the UK, where she was visiting to tell her mother that she was leaving Australia. She is now performing Indian head massage and hand massaging, but feels she could break out into hypnotherapy. Her limiting beliefs around her problem are certainly a thing of the past for Susie. Here is her story:

Susie had hypnotherapy for her bad knees. She hadn't really intended this to happen, but her daughter's belief in hypnotherapy was what brought about this wonderful transformation. Her knees had been giving her trouble for some years – she thought approximately 20 or more – and her daughter booked her into a hypnotherapy course, with the intention of convincing Susie that she could get rid of the pain through hypnotherapy. Susie was unaware of her daughter's intention. This is what she said about herself and her condition and, most of all, about her hypnotherapy:

My knees had been going downhill for a long time. I think that was for several reasons: my weight, it is a degenerative condition and it is also conditioning because my grandmother had terrible knees. My mother had a knee replacement, too, so I had an idea that it would be passed down to me. I don't dwell on things, though – my mother had macular degeneration and I don't have that. I do see now that maybe this thing with my knees could have been in my mind.

They were so bad that I couldn't go up the stairs. I could come down, but had to hang onto the bannisters. They just got progressively worse so I had one arthroscope, then a year or so later I had the other one done. At that time, they said they were ratchet and needed replacing; that was some 20 years ago. They told me that I would need knee replacements. I really didn't want that to happen. I never took any painkillers because I don't believe in them; all they do is mask the problem. My daughter always seemed to be annoyed about my inactivity and my knee problem, I think.

My daughter and I went to a weekend hypnotherapy seminar to learn something about hypnotherapy, and we met Shane and Jess. They were professional and not only was the content of the weekend great, but I got a good feeling about them. Their passion for what they were doing was amazing. I was beginning to think, 'I really like this hypnotherapy thing', not imagining that it would ever change my life!

My daughter was absolutely blown away by the possibilities of what hypnotherapy could do, and I must confess that I was too, even though if this had been back when I was younger that would not have been the case. You see, I was brought up in a very strict Catholic household and from a very early age believed in God and that prayer was the only solution – you would pray and that was it. I think this is why, when my daughter suggested that we go and do the next 5-day course, in Queensland, I agreed. For some reason, I really believed in Shane and Jess.

By the time we went to Queensland, just a few weeks after our initial weekend course, my knees were so bad that I was having to sit down after every few metres of walking, holding onto walls and begging my daughter to not make me walk. The pain was terrible.

At the course, many people were chosen to go up on stage with Shane to be hypnotised for all manner of problems as the course went through certain techniques. I was one of them. I felt a little sceptical, even though I trusted Shane completely. He asked how much of a problem was this problem of mine? Well, of course, I had to say 10 out of 10. It was holding me back in so many ways in where I went, how I felt, and it affected my family time so much.

After Shane had finished, I didn't really feel any different at first. I got up and walked off, but my knees felt just the same. It wasn't until after we finished the very long session (about 7 or 8 hours without a break) that I got up and almost ran to the lift. I didn't even think about it, or my knees. It was almost as if the problem had never existed! That day (oh yes, we hadn't finished for the day) when we went back for the second part of the session, I just forgot about them. I actually slept too, which I hadn't done for many years as the pain had been excruciating.

This course changed my life in so many ways. I still do not think that I am completely free of the restrictions I have put on myself, but I am certainly a long way to getting there. I also know that if I need further help with other things in the future like my weight, for instance, I can turn to hypnotherapy. My weight still holds me back to some degree, but I am willing to work on that, for sure. As for my knees, it has now been five months, and although if I sit too long they become a bit stiff or some days they ache a bit, I do not stress about them. They do not restrict the things I can do, and I sleep every night, without pain. I do not need medication, I do not need to think about an operation, which is a weight lifted off my shoulders, and I am now going to do the next course in hypnotherapy next month. It runs for a week and I can hardly wait. Bring it on, world!

What Susie's daughter said about Susie's transformation:

My mother's life changed and so did our whole family's after her transformation. Before hypnotherapy, my mother just wouldn't go anywhere, making excuses because of her knees. We were limited on holidays, outings, etc. Since her transformation, my mother walks for long distances and can stand for long lengths of time without complaint at all. She even went to Bali on a family holiday recently and joined in with every activity. It was fantastic to have her there and being a part of everything. It has truly changed all our lives.

Teneil's story

Profile: ICU Nurse, aged 32, married with one child (at time of hypnotherapy session)

I was having a terrible time when I heard Benetta say that she was practising hypnotherapy. You see, my child was almost three years old and we had been trying to have another baby for a year or so. Getting pregnant wasn't such a problem, but staying pregnant was. I didn't think it was such a big problem after the first miscarriage, but after the second and then the third, I had almost convinced myself that it just wasn't going to happen.

I had become so stressed about the whole thing that just the mention of babies or someone else becoming pregnant made me stressed and even angry. I felt terrible and would just go home and cry. Mentally, I was a mess about the whole thing. I just couldn't be happy for anyone else at that time.

I asked Benetta if she had ever helped anyone to either get pregnant or to deal with this anxiety I was feeling. She said that the anxiety was easy, and that she didn't see why it couldn't work. I had already booked into a fertility clinic but decided to give hypnotherapy a go. I mean, what did I have to lose?

In the first session we had, I just sat and told Benetta the whole story about the three miscarriages I'd had recently and about my feelings and anxiety centred around other people becoming pregnant, about myself becoming pregnant and, of course, carrying the baby to term.

Benetta made a connection between my first pregnancy being such a bad experience and my inability to carry a second child to term. Was it something that I had said to myself and believed, that I never wanted to have the whole problem of having another baby? I had been ill throughout the first pregnancy and during the later part had a car accident and ended up in hospital. I remember it vividly. Whilst we were discussing these things, I remembered saying to myself, 'Never again … I never want to do this again. It is far too traumatic.' Benetta said that when thinking of what to tell me during hypnosis, she actually included the fact that we do not always mean the things that we think and say to ourselves during times of trauma.

She also helped me greatly with the anxiety. I was given a mindfulness type of coping mechanism, to just deep breathe, centre myself and the anxiety would pass. This helped me tremendously, in particular when wondering if my baby was growing well and strong. (Oh yes, by the way, I became pregnant within two months of having the hypnotherapy, without even really trying.)

I also remembered odd things that were said to me whilst under hypnosis that also made me feel at ease. There was an analogy made between my growing baby and growing a flower in the greenhouse. Once pregnant again, if I didn't feel my baby move for a day or two, I would just think, 'Everything in the greenhouse is fine; my plant is growing.' Even though I did sometimes have seconds when I thought of the miscarriages I'd had, I still felt a sort of calm feeling and a strange knowledge that everything was going to be okay from now on.

As to how the hypnotherapy felt … well, it was different to how I'd thought it would feel. The only exposure I had had previously was seeing how it was done on the television. Things being dangled in front of someone and then them seemingly going so deeply into hypnosis that they flopped all over the place and seemed not to know what was happening. This could not have been further from the way it happened.

I sat down at Benetta's house (she still didn't have her office at that time) on a comfortable couch. Her dogs were around and there were all the normal noises going on. She put on some soothing background music and as I closed my eyes she started talking to me. I remember that I relaxed so easily, and my arms were sort of heavy. Then much of the next 40 minutes seemed to pass by so quickly I could have sworn it was only a few minutes. I really couldn't remember too much about the content of the things that were being said.

When I was brought back to full consciousness, I felt happy, relaxed and calm. I went home and nothing much seemed to have happened, but as the time went on I just seemed to not be thinking so much about the baby thing. It was about a week or so later when what would normally have set my anxiety off happened. A friend of mine said she was pregnant, but instead of the anxiety it previously would have caused, I actually felt happy and delighted for her. I really don't know why but it was a great feeling to not feel that anxiety. I think if you asked my husband, he would say that I was very different even though I really didn't feel that different within myself.

My pregnancy went without a hitch and even the birth was a dream. My darling little girl was born and she really is a dream child. Everyone comments on how much she smiles and how forward she is – so unlike my first pregnancy and first child. I know that every child is different and that the second child often seems to be easier to deal with, but I also think that it could be to do with how relaxed I was throughout my pregnancy and delivery.

I totally believe in the power of hypnotherapy and have recommended it to many of my friends since.

***

I had known Teneil for some time but had never really discussed the pregnancy problem with her. When she heard that I was a hypnotherapist, she asked me if I thought it would help her. When she said that she had already had three miscarriages and was looking at doing IVF, I said that I thought it would be good to try. As I have said before, I really want hypnotherapy to be the first thing people try, and this was no exception. IVF is not only a very involved and complex procedure but also very expensive, and so I was happy to try and so was Teneil.

One of the things I first addressed was the anxiety issue. I could see that she was having a lot of problems with this side of things, and if she achieved nothing else she was happy to be rid of the feelings she had around her pregnancy itself, and how unhappy she felt when her friends became pregnant. I just knew I could help her with this problem, but I also had a good feeling about her becoming pregnant and carrying her baby to term. As a therapist, you cannot give guarantees but you ultimately need to give hope. When Teneil left me, she already felt better – more relaxed and had the feeling that all would go well.

***

To finish off the story side of things, I just wanted to include a short story from a patient's wife. You see, even if they hadn't have thought of hypnotherapy during their search in the holistic world of treatments, then maybe they should have. I wish that I had been their first line of holistic treatment. However, to have been there to help with Theo's anguish and pain was an experience I will not forget.

Here is Tina and Theo's story:

Theo was diagnosed with renal cell carcinoma in April, 2014 at the age of 44. Within one month of being diagnosed, a radical nephrectomy was performed on his right kidney. The good news was that the 10cm tumour was contained to the kidney. It hadn't spread to any other parts of his body, so that would be the end of that ... or so that's what the surgeon said at one of our first consults.

After the surgery, the surgeon suggested that Theo do a course of chemotherapy because he had dropped pieces of the tumour in Theo's abdomen. He explained this as 'precautionary measure' but he was sure he had removed all that the eye could see ...

The oncologist prescribed Theo with a course of oral chemotherapy, which he would take once a day for six months. This made Theo very unwell at times, with side effects such as nausea, tiredness, vision difficulties and many more. But throughout the whole course, Theo would get up and go to work every morning to set up his boys, as he had his own rendering business. He trained at the gym at least four times a week and was a very committed dad to our three beautiful daughters and their weekly activities. Theo also loved martial arts and even completed his Black Belt 1st Dan in Jujitsu while he was on chemo.

We could never really understand how *Theo* could get cancer. Strong, fit, healthy, young are the words that come to mind when you would look at him. Theo remembered his father always being sick on the couch (high blood pressure and strokes). He never wanted this for his daughters so made it a priority to be fit and healthy. Goes to show cancer does not discriminate. For Theo, it was business as usual and he just did what he had to do, no complaining and always with a smile. I just knew he would be fine so I really wasn't worried.

December, 2014, chemo finally finished, we got our scan results and *no more cancer*! Best news ever … Good-bye and good riddance to 2014 and hello, 2015 – to bigger and better things in our lives. We could finally move on as the last couple of years had been hell: our house had flooded and six weeks after that burned to the ground; fighting with insurance; renting a two bedroom unit; the cancer … it was enough to send us off the edge but it didn't. The love and commitment to each other and our girls made us stronger as a family.

So, 2015 was going to be our year … but it definitely did not turn out how we had planned. In February, 2015, Theo's cancer came back, this time in the lining of the abdomen: peritoneal carcinomatosis. I remember asking the oncologist, 'So, what stage is it at?' He replied, '4.' I knew that was not good. I remember holding Theo's hand and we were both in shock. The prognosis was absolutely devastating. I honestly thought Theo had beaten this; how could it come back?

Not much was offered to Theo as treatment, but more to prolong his life rather than a cure. We walked out of the hospital just gutted, and for the next couple of days we were on a roller coaster ride of emotions. Once Theo got his head around what the next step was, it was business as usual. He was not the type to dwell. I was also trying to be positive but, just quietly, I was a mess and could not get past the fact that my husband had a terminal illness and he was not going to be around for me and our girls.

This time around, Theo decided to go for alternative treatment as opposed to chemo again, as the chemo didn't work the first time. He was willing to give anything a go if it meant he would live. I supported Theo with whatever choices he made regarding his treatment. After lots of research, homeopaths, naturopaths, diet changes, organic everything and a con artist who claimed he has cured cancer, Theo was adamant this was going to work for him. Theo kept positive throughout this whole process, whereas I was very overwhelmed with all of the new information, trying to keep all our lives as normal as possible and holding the fort without crumbling.

Our final family holiday was in July and we had an amazing time in Thailand. Once we came back, Theo celebrated his 45th birthday with our immediate families. Theo had not seen a doctor since March, so we never really knew where we were at, and I know Theo didn't want to know.

We ended up at the Austin Emergency, where scans confirmed the tumours had grown with new tumours contained to the abdomen and it was pretty much downhill from there. From draining ascites every couple of weeks, blood transfusions fortnightly, immunotherapy every three weeks, rapid weight loss, occasional hospital stays and the poking and prodding … this was the last three months of his life. It was all too much for Theo at times – physically and mentally – and I could see he just wanted a break. It absolutely killed me seeing him in so much pain.

The final week, it all just happened far too quickly. I really thought he was coming home with me. I knew I was losing him and I could not do a damn thing to save him, but I sat next to him, holding his hand the whole time; it's all I could do. It's the comfort he wanted and needed. At times, he was calm and relaxed and at others he felt agitated and anxious. This is where Benetta came into the picture and did her beautiful work on Theo, helping him to relax and to even visualise himself being at home with his daughters and myself. I just loved seeing him happy, even if it was temporary. I know it really helped him during that awful time.

For Theo, he was more concerned about his four girls, even when he was at his worst. Theo and I met in 1993 and married in 2000. Our family, for us, was perfect; Theo and I were perfect for each other. We have three beautiful daughters: Marie, 15, Deana, 12 and Alexandra, 8. He was our *hero*; our lives have changed forever.

Throughout his journey, Theo was always focused on what needed to be done to get better. He never wanted to accept that this disease had finally taken him down. He fought till the end … November 17, 2015.

***

I met Theo and Tina when Theo was ill so I wasn't lucky enough to know how vibrant he was prior to his illness. What I do know is that he never, ever complained. He was stoic and loving, and anyone could see just the sort of person he was.

On the night that I helped him with some relaxation and visualisation, he was in pain, both physically and mentally. His anguish at having to leave his beautiful family was taking its toll on him as well as Tina. We all sat together and I asked him, 'Where would you like to be?' He said, 'At home with the kids and Tina.' So, as I helped him to relax and to forget about his disease, we also visualised him at home with his family, just sitting, watching them play and laugh.

I know it helped, and I know that I can help so many people like Theo; people just don't know that. I wished that I'd have known earlier that he was trying all those natural therapies so that I could have helped sooner. I may not have been able to help him cure himself, but maybe I could have. We will never know now, but to anyone who wants to try, I am here. I really hope that in the future I can help Tina and her children, too, to see what a privilege it was for me to be a tiny part of Theo's life, and that his family should all feel that the time spent with such a man is marvellous. Many thanks for sharing this story with everyone, Tina.

Chapter 7
Conclusion

In conclusion, I would like to thank all my clients, family and friends who have told their stories to help me to try and help others. As far as I am concerned, the only evidence I have and can give to you to help you decide if hypnotherapy can help you is these stories. They are true, and sometimes raw, and if those people can achieve those things, why not you, too?

In my office, I do not like the word 'can't'. What I do like is, 'How can we?' 'How can we find a solution to the problem?' is a much better fit. I never say, 'Never'; I always say, 'Let us see how we can.' Often I see the solution straight away; however, if the problem is complicated it may take a few meetings for us to completely solve the problem. It is always up to the client, though. How deep do they want to go, how much time and money do they want to spend? I will always do my best, as I know my colleagues from other states will do.

If you are not local to Melbourne, then I can offer consultations via Skype, write a session for you that you can listen to at home, or refer you to another hypnotherapist in most states in Australia. I have many connections with my hypno-family. If you feel you would like to give it a try, you can contact me via the email addresses contained at the back of the book.

Please, do not live a life filled with regret, fear or beliefs that restrict you. Live life the best way you can. Maybe you, too, will then believe in miracles (whatever interpretation you may give that statement) as I do.

I really hope that you have enjoyed reading and learning a little more about my profession and my passion. Many thanks for buying this book and taking time out to read it.

About the Author

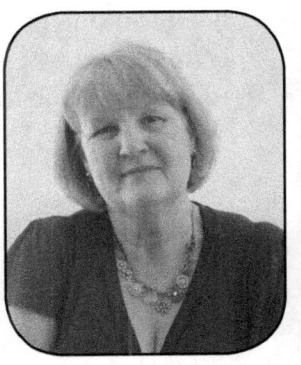

Benetta grew up in a small English town, Kettering. After finishing school, she went on to technical college for three years and then started to train as a lawyer. She hated it and decided to look into nursing as a profession after it was suggested she had the right attitude for dealing with people. Benetta loved her nurse training from the start and nursed in several different fields in the UK. She later went to Saudi Arabia, where she met her husband, Derek.

Benetta and Derek went back to the UK and, after finding it difficult to settle there, decided to move to Australia in 1994 with their two children, aged eleven months and two-and-a-half years at the time.

During the past few years, Benetta had been thinking of making a move from nursing into something more holistic. She discovered hypnotherapy and found it to be just the right fit for her. Opening her own business was daunting, but is the best thing she has ever done.

Benetta now resides in the northern suburbs of Melbourne and although she has worked in many fields during her nursing career, had been working on an oncology ward for the past eighteen years before deciding to make the move toward working in hypnotherapy full-time.

Special Offer

I hope you enjoyed reading this short but sweet book. It is now time to find out if that miracle can be yours too! I really want everyone to try hypnotherapy to help them solve their problem, so I am offering a special to you, my reader.

You can book a 1-hour session for $75 (normally valued at $150) at my office in Diamond Creek, 3089, or over the internet if this is more convenient. This session will cover your initial interview, and we may be able to resolve your problem, or at least make a start.

You can book your session by contacting me on 0418 126 811. If you are still unsure about the process I am willing to do a 5-minute consultation over the phone, where I will be happy to see if we can work together.

I look forward to meeting with you!

Recommended Practitioners

Below I have included my contact details and a list of other practitioners who offer particular services or who live interstate. Some of these practitioners have gone further than hypnotherapy and include other holistic advanced therapies or specialise in certain therapies such as dealing with life-changing conditions, or parenting and relationship problems.

Benetta Wainman
Road to Success Hypnotherapy
Master Hypnotherapist, NLP and Timeline Transformation
Melbourne, VIC
0418 126 811
benettaw1@gmail.com
roadtosuccesshypnotherapy.com

Helen Antoniou
R&R Wellness
Master Hypnotherapist, NLP and Timeline Transformation
Adelaide, SA
0477 164 783
facebook.com/RRWellnessRejuvenate

Ruby Bell
The Empowered Self
Master Hypnotherapist and Certified Clinical Hypnotherapist
0426 881 896
theempoweredself@mail.com
theempoweredself.org

Morgana Boerner
The Avalon Touch
Parenting and Relationship Coach
Geelong, VIC
0423 383 598
morgana@theavalontouch.com.au
theavalontouch.com.au

Helen Bolger-Harris
Unlimited in Life
Business and Life Mindset Productivity for Women
Carnegie, VIC
0428 744 048
admin@helenbolgerharris.com
helenbolgerharris.com

Karine Chalmers
Beauty and Body Care
Master Hypnotherapist, NLP and Timeline Transformation
Sydney, NSW
0413 494 712
karine@aushypnosis.com
beautyandbodycare.com

Joy Fairhall
Mind, Body, Joy
Specialist in emotional support and Guidance Coach for people with life-changing illness
Doncaster East, VIC
0403 224 134
joy@mindbodyjoy.com.au
mindbodyjoy.com.au

Indira Hnatiuk
Elemental Drives
Master Hypnotherapist, NLP and EFT. BSc in Chinese Medicine and Life Coach
Macquarie, ACT
0466 437 857
facebook.com/ElementalDrives

Lashay Hole
Extreme You
Master Practitioner Hypnotherapist
Shepparton, VIC
0401 878 951
facebook.com/Extreme-You

Susie Mornement
Master Hypnotherapist and NLP Practitioner
Albury, NSW
0422 455 365

Adaire Palmer
Master Hypnotherapist and NLP Practitioner
Adelaide, SA
0408 792 762
adaires01@yahoo.com
adairepalmer.com.au

Emma Romano
Master Hypnotherapist, NLP Practitioner and Energy Healer
Albury, NSW
0423 119 045
emma@emmaromano.com.au
emmaromano.com.au

Tracie Taft
Empowered Directions
Hypnotherapist and Mindset Coach
Rowville, VIC
0481 304 440
tracie@empowereddirections.com
empowereddirections.com

For hypnotherapy training or courses in Relationship Success or World Class Speaker Training, contact:

Shane and Jess Fozard
Australian Success Academy
0468 399 468
support@australiansuccess.com
australiansuccess.com
Shane and Jess Fozard, founders of Australian Success Academy and the Australian Hypnosis Certification, run arguably Australia's #1 most positive and supportive Hypnosis and mindset related communities in Australia, if not the world.

Shane and Jess

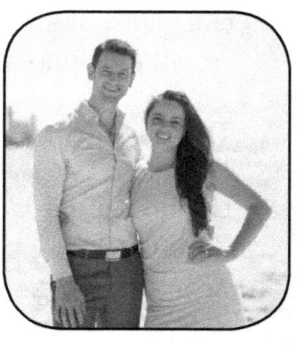

*H*aving trained thousands of business owners, therapists, executives, parents and students through their live certification programs, Shane and Jess provide not only the education and information on what hypnosis is and how to use it, but more importantly, they deliver a highly-engaging and deeply-transformational experience throughout each of their programs.

As each graduate of their introductory and advanced courses can attest to, Australian Success Academy prides itself on delivering value as well as providing ongoing support to ensure each participant gets real world results.

To discover more about Australian Success Academy and their programs, go to www.australiansuccess.com.

Adair

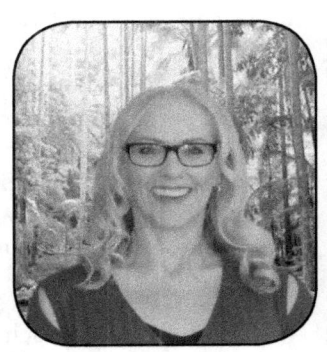

*B*enetta and I met in October 2015 when we both decided to do the Neuro Linguistic Programmming (NLP) course after successfully completing the Hypnotherapy Certification course with the Australian Success Academy early in the year. Benetta did her certification in Melbourne and I did mine in Adelaide. The NLP course was being held on the Gold Coast. We shared accommodation for the duration of the course and formed a strong friendship.

We are both practicing hypnotherapists, Benetta in Victoria, and myself in South Australia and now taking the practice online, where I can help more people from further afield. We have plans in the future to expand and run group sessions and workshops together too!

Hypnotherapy for me was like a lightning bolt of inspiration as I was struggling with issues of self-confidence and addictions. I was a heavy smoker and drinker and also had 'food fights' with myself regularly. All pointing towards a continued downward spiral, particularly as I was quite good at blaming other people for what was happening to me. I thought I was taking responsibility for my life, but in reality, I was shifting it all to those who 'did me wrong'.

Less than 3 weeks after doing the Hypnotherapy Certification course, I threw away the cigarettes and have never looked back. I've also eliminated alcohol from my diet and have made friends with the food in my life. Relationships are also better as I feel better and better about who I am and begin to understand the true power of living a life that is on purpose and at cause. 'At cause' is a term I learnt doing the hypnotherapy training and I believe it's the most powerful concept for people taking back control over their lives.

Becoming a practicing hypnotherapist felt like a dichotomy, both the next, natural step in my ongoing development and personal growth and also one of the most frightening things I have done (except public speaking, but I'm OK with that now, too). The responsibility of building rapport so strongly with others so I can help them as much as they need was a big hurdle at first. Then it became a more natural thing to do as I learnt more, practiced more and the shoes of the 'practicing hypnotherapist' started to feel quite good on me.

We each have a special gift (or gifts) to bring to the world, and it's near to impossible to bring those gifts and talents out unless we do work on ourselves to move past limiting beliefs and negative self-talk. Hypnotherapy is an amazing tool to help us do this and I'm blessed that it's been placed in my hands to help others with. I'm also blessed that Benetta and I have been able to walk this part of our lives journeys together to make a difference in the lives of others.

Joy

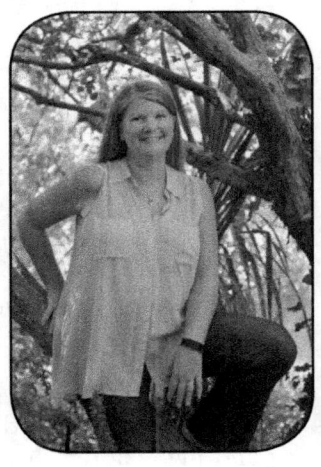

'Joy' is not a word you associate with at a time when you have been affected by a Life Changing diagnosis or event. At a time when your whole world feels like you've been sucked into a big black vortex of swirling emotions, fear, uncertainty and even grief. Your world, as you know it, has been changed forever and, not only your world but also the world of all those that love and care for you. Suddenly your identity, as you know it, your present and your future identity, has been changed forever.

Hypnosis, and other tools and techniques, certainly assist during times like these. On being diagnosed you may struggle to cope with your own emotions and there are the fears and associations surrounding illness, all these emotions respond well through hypnosis.

In my experience of working with those affected, the biggest emotion is fear – particularly fear of the unknown. The most common fearful questions are 'What if', 'How will I?', 'What happens if?', and 'Why me?', While a hypnotherapist can't answer these questions, we can assist you through your fears through hypnosis. Hypnosis, as Benetta has explained throughout this book, works with your subconscious to control and provide techniques to remove fears and provide you with the strength and ways to face those fears so you can focus on your health moving forward.

So why do I say Joy should be felt during times like these? By tapping what has bought you Joy, Happiness and Confidence in the past reduces the stress cortisol in your body providing a greater health benefit and optimum benefit for your health. So through hypnosis another benefit is a benefit for your mental state by feeling Joy and Happiness and thus reducing anxiety and distress.

I personally know, having lost my husband to cancer, that hypnosis assisted with my grief and gave me and my children the strength to move on into our new future, a future without their Dad and myself without my wonderful husband. Therefore, for these very personal reasons, why I studied and now practise hypnotherapy and why I'm so passionate about my work and supporting those who have been where I've been.

Joy Fairhall
Emotional Support and Guidance Coach
Mind Body Joy

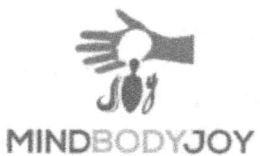

www.ingramcontent.com/pod-product-compliance
Lightning Source LLC
Chambersburg PA
CBHW070632300426
44113CB00010B/1747